EDITED BY HELEN EXLEY

Published in 2019 by Helen Exley® LONDON in Great Britain.
Illustration by Juliette Clarke © Helen Exley Creative Ltd 2019.
All the words by Dalton Exley, Odile Dormeuil, Pam Brown,
Charlotte Gray, Hannah C. Klein, Stuart & Linda Macfarlane,
Peter Gray, Mathilde and Sébastian Forestier, Pamela Dugdale
and Linda Gibson © Helen Exley Creative Ltd 2019.
Design, selection and arrangement © Helen Exley Creative Ltd 2019.
The moral right of the author has been asserted.

ISBN 978-1-78485-200-9

12 11 10 9 8 7 6 5 4 3 2 1

OTHER BOOKS IN THE SERIES

THE LITTLE BOOK OF *Gratitude*
THE LITTLE BOOK OF *Happiness*
THE LITTLE BOOK OF *Kindness*
THE LITTLE BOOK OF *Smiles*

Helen Exley® LONDON
16 Chalk Hill, Watford, Herts WD19 4BG, UK
www.helenexley.com

THE LITTLE BOOK OF

Hope

Helen Exley

If you can
dream it,
you can do it.

WALT DISNEY

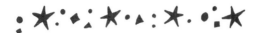

No matter how weary
or dreary you may feel,
you possess the certainty that…
absolutely anything may happen.
And the fact that it practically always
doesn't, matters not one jot.
The possibility is always there.

MONICA BALDWIN

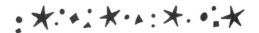

The tree which needs
two arms to span its girth
sprang from the tiniest shoot.
The tower, nine storeys high,
rose from a mound of earth.
A journey of a thousand miles
began with a single step.

LAO TZU

However long
the night,
the dawn
will break.

AFRICAN PROVERB

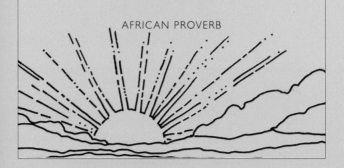

Every day
is an astounding gift.
Open each eagerly.

PAM BROWN

When I look
into the future,
it's so bright
it burns my eyes.

OPRAH WINFREY

Tomorrow is the most
important thing in life.
Comes into us at midnight
very clean. It's perfect
when it arrives
and it puts itself in our hands.

JOHN WAYNE

All our dreams and desires,
creations, plans
are fed by hope.

ODILE DORMEUIL

Hopeful as the
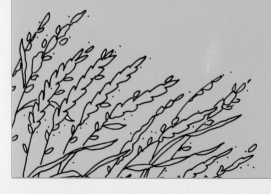

reak of day...

THOMAS BAILEY ALDRICH

Keep your face
to the sunshine
and you cannot
see the shadow.

HELEN KELLER
(BORN BOTH DEAF AND BLIND)

No monument.

No city.

No nation.

Nothing worthwhile

has ever been built

without hope.

STUART & LINDA MACFARLANE

There is no medicine like hope,

no incentive so great,

and no tonic so powerful

as expectation of something.

ORISON SWETT MARDEN

*True hope
is swift,
and flies
with swallow's
wings.*

WILLIAM SHAKESPEARE

A person can live
about forty days without food,
about three days
without water,
about eight minutes
without air,
but only for one second
without hope.

JOSEPH ADDISON

The earth is empty.
The trees, once thick with blossom
stand dead against a bitter sky.
The streams are frozen.
Hope is lost.
But see – along the branches
new buds appear and greenness
pushes through the ground unnoticed.
Spring may be slow –
but will at last return.

PAM BROWN

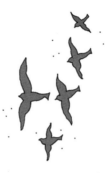

The birds of hope
are everywhere,
listen to them sing.

TERRI GUILLEMETS

Hope is the poor

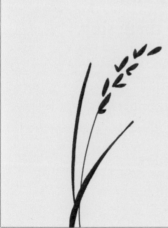

...person's bread.

GEORGE HERBERT

Hope – that marvellous ingredient
that keeps humanity going –
something that is almost as vital
to people as love...
belief in tomorrow,
bright expectations that refuse to die.

MARJORIE HOLMES

The best doctors
know how vital hope's role
is in many successful
patient recoveries.

DALTON EXLEY

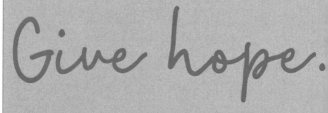

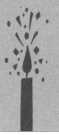

Without hope we cannot go on.
Without hope we cannot live.

DOROTHY DAY

When you cease to dream you cease to live.

MALCOLM S. FORBES

Give life.

PAMELA DUGDALE

Hope for love, success, security.
Adventure and discovery. Peace and joy.

ODILE DORMEUIL

To travel hopefully
is a better thing than to arrive.

ROBERT LOUIS STEVENSON

Freedom is hope -

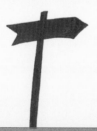

Hope can tear down prison walls.

STUART & LINDA MACFARLANE

ope is freedom.

MATHILDE AND SÉBASTIEN FORESTIER

I dream my painting,
then I paint my dream.

VINCENT VAN GOGH

Hope carries us,
soaring high above the driving
winds of life.

ANA JACOBS

How very different our lives
from the Sumerians,
Egyptians, Greeks and Romans.
And yet we share
the self-same legacy
of courage, love and hope.

PETER GRAY

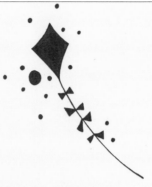

In the dark of winter
when everything seems dry and dead,
look more closely.
Almost invisible,
the first bright sparks of green
are coming through.
The promises of Spring.

CHARLOTTE GRAY

Spring in the world! And all things are made new.

WILLIAM BLAKE

Hope helps you
turn things around.
It helps you find
purpose and add reason
for all your hard work
and struggles.
Hope helps you,
hope's your friend.

DALTON EXLEY

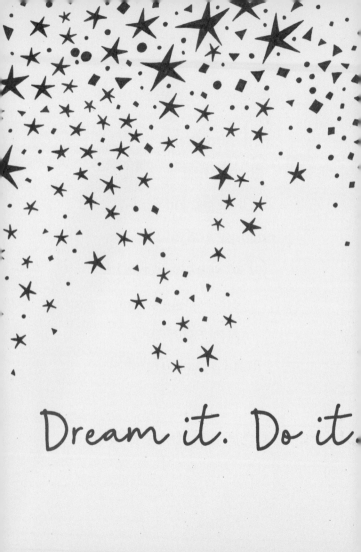

Dream it. Do it.

Hope is freedom –
it lets us live without the shackles
of worry and fear.

MATHILDE AND SÉBASTIEN FORESTIER

Hope, child, tomorrow
and tomorrow still,
And every tomorrow hope;
trust while you live.

VICTOR HUGO

ive in Hope.

LINDA MACFARLANE

Look up!
Look up
and make a wish.
May it
come true!

PAM BROWN

Hope helps us stand when sadness threatens to buckle us.
Hope restores our energy when circumstances seem to defeat us.
Hope glorifies the mundane.
Hope gives us the courage to dare to be ourselves and to reveal ourselves to others.
To live in hope is to believe in light when it is dark, in beauty when ugliness abounds, in peace when conflict seems to reign.

SUZANNE C. COLE

I live a day at a time.

Each day I look for a kernel

of excitement.

In the morning,

I say:

"What is my exciting thing for today?"

Then, I do the day.

Don't ask me about tomorrow.

BARBARA JORDAN

At the end of the day,
each of us has very different opportunities,
but we all have the right to a better life –
the right to dream,
the right to hope.

DAME KELLY HOLMES

Live hopefully.
It does not matter what happens,
what your circumstances are,
you have something to connect with.

BEAR HEART (MUSKOGEE)

Hope is renewed with every sunrise.

ODILE DORMEUIL

In the depth
of winter,
I finally learned
that within me
there lay an
invincible summer.

ALBERT CAMUS

Our lives are small,
our dreams are great.
We live with faith and hope
in the small corners of our days.

KENT NERBURN

We have enough people
who tell it like it is –
now we could use a few
who tell it like it can be.

ROBERT ORBEN

May you always find new roads
to travel; new horizons to explore;
new dreams to call your own.

MARK ORTMAN

Hope is the pillar
that holds up
the world.

PLINY THE ELDER

No pessimist ever discovered
the secrets of the stars, or sailed
to an uncharted land, or opened
a new heaven to the human spirit.

HELEN KELLER
(BORN BOTH DEAF AND BLIND)

I dwell in

H ope may seem a frail
and vulnerable thing,
but it can be stronger than steel if harnessed
with courage and determination.

DALTON EXLEY

Hope doesn't die in winter, hope grows in winter. It's the most difficult circumstances of life, the winter seasons of life, that give rise to the strongest hope.

WOODROW KROLL

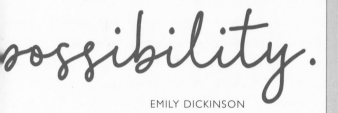

possibility.

EMILY DICKINSON

When your head
is pounding
and your heart is
thumping
and your legs are jelly
hope can still
get you across
the finishing line.

PAM BROWN

Light is stronger than darkness.
Hold on to light.
Let it strengthen you.

TERRY WAITE

Hope inspires determination,
Hope inspires bravery,
Hope inspires sacrifice.
Through hope miracles
have been performed
by ordinary people.

MATHILDE AND SÉBASTIEN FORESTIER

Stars over snow,
And in the west a planet
Swinging below a star –
Look for a lovely thing
and you will find it,
It is not far –
It never will be far.

SARA TEASDALE

Far away there in the sunshine
are my highest aspirations.
I may not reach them,
but I can look up and see their beauty,
believe in them…

LOUISA MAY ALCOTT

Our way is not
soft grass, it's
a mountain path
with lots of rocks.
But it goes upwards,
forward, toward
the sun.

DR. RUTH WESTHEIMER

Hope is the silver thread
that guides us through the dark.

PAM BROWN

When you've dreamt of something,
hoped beyond hope for it for so long,
you can't even remember
how long, hope finally brings you
unmatched joy.

DALTON EXLEY

Each time we smell

the autumn's

dying scent,

We know that

primrose time

will come again.

SAMUEL TAYLOR COLERIDGE

Often people have a tragic story to tell –
but rather than let adversity
be a burden they let it become an
inspiration to others in similar
circumstances.
These people who find hope –
even in tragedy and, turn tragedy
into hope.

STUART & LINDA MACFARLANE

Hope seems frail
but has the
strength of steel.

PAMELA DUGDALE

There is always in February some one day,
at least, when one smells the yet distant,
but surely coming summer.
Perhaps it is a warm, mossy scent
that greets one when passing along
the southern side of a hedge-bank;
or it may be in some woodland opening,
where the sun has coaxed out the
pungent smell of the trailing ground ivy,
whose blue flowers will soon appear;
but the day always comes, and with it
the glad certainty that summer is nearing
and that the good things promised
will never fail.

GERTRUDE JEKYLL

My heart stands
in waiting and hope
as the trees stand still
through the darkness
of night.

HAZRAT INAYAT KHAN

Hold on to hope.
It seems so frail a thing
– but it will keep your head
above the water
while you find a foothold
and achieve the shore.
It's there just ahead.
So don't give in.
Firm ground and reassurance.
Waiting for you.

PAM BROWN

If one is lucky,
a single fantasy
can transform
a million realities.

MAYA ANGELOU

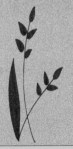

Without hope
the human race
would have perished
long ago.

CHARLOTTE GRAY

Hope is a wal

Aid-workers bring shelter,
food, medicines
– and, the most vital thing of all,
hope.

ODILE DORMEUIL

ng dream.

ARISTOTLE

To hope means to be ready at every moment for that which is not yet born, and yet not become desperate if there is no birth in our lifetime. Those whose hope is weak settle for comfort or for violence, those whose hope is strong see and cherish signs of new life and are ready every moment to help the birth of that which is ready to be born.

ERICH FROMM

To live in utter poverty,
to create meals from almost nothing,
to keep the children clothed and safe,
to bring laughter into dreariness,
to keep hope alive
– this is true, enduring hope and courage.

PAM BROWN

Life is a pure flame,
and we live by an invisible sun
within us.

SIR THOMAS BROWNE

Hope begins in the dark,
the stubborn hope that if you
just show up and try to
do the right thing,
the dawn will come.
You wait and watch and work:
you don't give up.

ANNE LAMOTT

Hope is a seed - tend

LINDA GIBSON

There are three things I was born
with in this world,
and there are three things
I will have until the day I die:
hope,
determination,
and song.

MIRIAM MAKEBA

t, care for it.

Happiness may pass –
but it will come again.
Certain as springtime follows winter.
As sun comes after rain.

ODILE DORMEUIL

Hope can make the present moment
less difficult to bear.
If we believe that tomorrow will be better,
we can bear a hardship today.

THICH NHAT HANH

Hope, I realized now, was irrepressible…
It welled up naturally in response
to fear and uncertainty, returning again
and again, like a living thing.

MARIA HOUSDEN

Hold your head high,
stick your chest out.
You can make it.
It gets dark sometimes
but morning comes…

JESSE JACKSON

Most of the important things
in the world have been accomplished
by people who have kept on trying
when there seemed to be no hope at all.

DALE CARNEGIE

When one door is shut,
another opens.

MIGUEL DE CERVANTES

When the well runs dry,
all that is left is hope.
When the harvest fails,
all that is left is hope.
When a child must beg on the streets,
all that is left is hope.
For many in this world
all they have left is hope…
hope and your love.

STUART & LINDA MACFARLANE

Of all the forces
that make for a better world,
none is so indispensable,
none so powerful, as hope.
Without hope people are only half alive.
With hope they dream
and think and work.

CHARLES SAWYER

Somewhere, something incredible
is waiting to be known.

CARL SAGAN

Isn't it nice to think that tomorrow is a new day with no mistakes in it yet?

LUCY MAUD MONTGOMERY

If you lose hope,
somehow you lose the vitality
that keeps moving,
you lose that courage to be,
that quality that helps you
go on in spite of it all.

MARTIN LUTHER KING JR.

Allow hope to penetrate
your darkness
and it will give you comfort.
And strength. And patience.

PAMELA DUGDALE

The poor person who has hope possesses more than any millionaire.

PAM BROWN

A life without hope
of any sort was no life:
it was a sky without stars,
a landscape of sorrow and emptiness.

ALEXANDER MCCALL SMITH

If you have hoped
and your expectation was not fulfilled
then go on hoping.

THE TALMUD

Sad soul, take comfort, nor forget
That sunrise never failed us yet.

CELIA THAXTER

The world is round and the place
which may seem like the end may also
be the beginning.

IVY BAKER PRIEST

Dreamers are artists,
poets and musicians.
Dreamers are accountants,
engineers and plumbers.
A dreamer is anyone
who is willing to make tomorrow
a little better than today.

STUART & LINDA MACFARLANE

Nothing is impossible...
Because nothing
is impossible,
you have to dream
big dreams;
the bigger,
the better.

MICHAEL PHELPS

Hope ever urges on,
and tells us tomorrow will be better.

TIBULLUS

Hope and courage
can bring an end to slavery,
Hope and courage
can bring equality for everyone,
Hope and courage
can bring freedom from cruel dictators,
What will your
hope and courage bring?

MATHILDE AND SÉBASTIEN FORESTIER

When the world
says, "Give up"
Hope whispers,
"Try it
one more time."

AUTHOR UNKNOWN

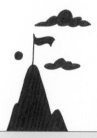

If you come to a thing
with no preconceived notions
of what that thing is,
the whole world can be your canvas.
Just dream it,
and you can make it so.

WHOOPI GOLDBERG

Hope is like a road in the country;
there was never a road,
but when many people walk on it,
the road comes into existence.

LIN YUTANG

We are all on this sea together.
But the lighthouse
is always there,
ready to show us the way home.

CHRISTOPHER REEVE

Those who have been deprived
of everything
by war and famine, flood and fire,
need shelter, food and water,
and a little hope.

PAM BROWN

...misfortune and destruction
are not final.
When the grass has been burnt
by the fire of the steppe,
it will grow anew in summer.

MONGOLIAN WISDOM

It isn't a calamity
to die with dreams unfulfilled,
but it is a calamity
not to dream…

BENJAMIN MAYS

I inhale hope
with every breath
I take.

SHARON PENMAN

There is nothing worth achieving
that can't be achieved,
There is nothing worth doing
that can't be done,
No mountain too high,
no ocean too deep,
If you just have hope.

STUART & LINDA MACFARLANE

Once you choose hope,
anything is possible.

CHRISTOPHER REEVE

In our moments of anguish,
gates barred for ever seem to open
and let in many a flood of light.

SWAMI VIVEKANANDA

In the hour of adversity
be not without hope,
for crystal rain
falls from black clouds.

PERSIAN PROVERB

W e are all in the gutter,
but some of us
are looking at the stars.

OSCAR WILDE

I think that wherever your journey
takes you there are new gods
waiting there,
with divine patience – and laughter.

SUSAN M. WATKINS

Hope is
the enemy
of defeat.

WOODROW KROLL

Do not stand at the foot

of a mountain and say,

"That is impossible".

Stand at the top

and say,

"Nothing is impossible".

STUART & LINDA MACFARLANE

Everything that is done in the world

is done by hope.

MARTIN LUTHER

There is no greater heroism
than loving and caring
after all hope is gone.

CHARLOTTE GRAY

Believe in hope, grow into hope,
and breathe in at every moment
the fragrance and beauty of hope.

SRI CHINMOY

When it is dark enough,
you can see the stars.

RALPH WALDO EMERSON

Remembering that you are going to die
is the best way I know to avoid
the trap of thinking you have something
to lose. You are already naked.
There is no reason not to follow your heart.

STEVE JOBS

To live without hope
is to cease to live.

FYODOR MIKHAILOVICH DOSTOYEVSKY

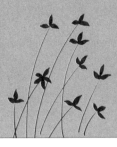

Hope's such a wonderful thing!
Helping humanity through the ages,
now and into the future.
Bright hope shines within all of us.
Believe in it, believe in yourself,
believe in today.

DALTON EXLEY

When you push a bulb deep
into soft wet soil, it is always
a symbol of hope – hope that you nature
will not fail; hope that you will still be alive
to see the bulb burst out of the ground
and unfurl its delicate leaves,
opening the way for the flower.
It is about a future you can only
hope for: maybe you won't see the flower
in all its glory, but someone will.

ROSIE BOYCOTT

What is a
person finally
left with?

Hope.

DIOGENES

✳ ✳ ✳

We must accept
finite
disappointment,
but we must never
lose infinite hope.

MARTIN LUTHER KING JR.

In the midst of the direst poverty
and despair, the human spirit,
especially that of children,
will find some hope to cling to,
some promise of a better day.

DOLLY PARTON

The miserable have no other medicine,
but only hope.

WILLIAM SHAKESPEARE

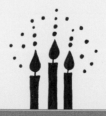

Fears cast long shadows that stretch out
way beyond their measure.
But fears can be vanquished with hope.

STUART & LINDA MACFARLANE

Learning to hope well is a small,
quiet, subtle thing –
but something that accumulates
day by day into an unstoppable force.

STEPHEN BOWKETT

In our struggles we may think
we can't go any further,
not realizing that it is merely
a turning point in our life.
All power is available to us.
You can turn things around
in your own life,
live hopefully,
and keep that hope going.

BEAR HEART (MUSKOGEE)

When the storm passes, the grasses will rise up again.

AFRICAN PROVERB

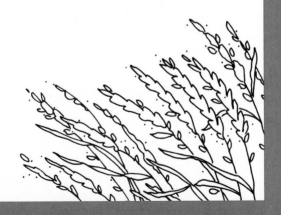

The first sparrow
of spring!
The year
beginning with
younger hope
than ever!

HENRY DAVID THOREAU

Winter is on
my head,
but eternal

spring
is in my heart.

VICTOR HUGO